10 Easy Exercises for a Perfectly Toned Body in a Month

LEGAL NOTES

ISBN-13: 978-1523433667

ISBN-10: 1523433663

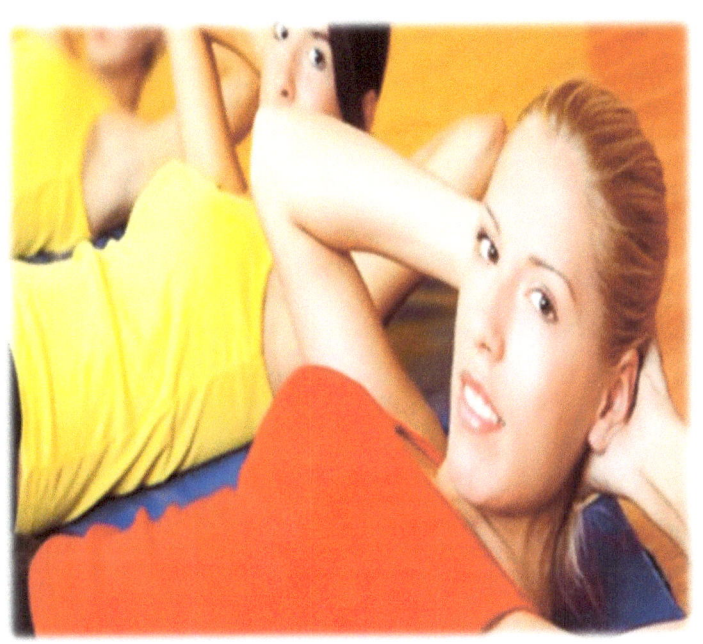

INTRODUCTION

Whether it is love handles, tire tubes, cellulite, or those other tricky trouble zones, the worst nightmare of every woman these days is to live with these and maintain a hectic routine while balancing work and home. As a matter of fact, almost every woman has to cross this unwanted phase in her life. It's time to stop wondering about how those fit women stay in shape with gorgeously toned bodies even after pregnancy and not spending too much time in the gym. Just fasten up for a little extra work to tighten up and tone your body for a daily 30-minute easy workout. We have gathered a solid set of moves that can help you shape up and feel confident in your favorite dresses.

Get in shape without any hassle with these top 10 toning exercises that can work wonders for your stomach, inner thighs, hips, waist, and shoulders. Read on to find out how you can add them into your workout routine.

TABLE OF CONTENTS

Introduction 4

Get Ready! 1

EXERCISE 1. Crunches 2

EXERCISE 2.Side Crunches 5

EXERCISE 3.Best Lower Abdomen Toning Exercise 8

EXERCISE 4.Gaining Back the Trimmed Curves 11

EXERCISE 5.Upper Body Toning 14

EXERCISE 6.Bench Press 18

EXERCISE 7.Push-Ups 21

EXERCISE 8.Chair Crunch 23

EXERCISE 9.Squat Thrust 25

EXERCISE 10.Dead Bug 28

Bonus Topics
10 things to do for an ache-free workout 30

Conclusion 35

Other Books By The Author. 36

Can I Ask A Favor? 38

GET READY!

Things you need

- A comfortable corner of your home or workplace where you can spare 30 minutes and do your workout without disturbance

- Small chair

- Dumbbells or water bottles

- Resistance or exercise band

Warm-up

These toning exercises should be set according to your recommended weekly target for strength. Always begin with a 6-minute warm-up and end with a 5-minute stretch and cool down routine – it's essential to avoid any strain in your muscles and to maintain a regular heart rate. For warming up, you can start by marching in place for 2 minutes and going into a light jog for 1 minute. This will help your heart rate and blood rush to your muscles to make them ready for the workout.

EXERCISE 1.

Crunches

T he first place where all the excessive fats get stored in your body is your tummy. Whether it is due to bad eating habits, hormonal imbalances, an always-sitting office job, pregnancy and post-delivery flab, or any other reason, your tummy muscles have to bear the consequences on the very first note. Abdominal crunches are proven for toning up your tummy and tucking it back. Only 5 minutes of this simple and easy exercise can do wonders for your abdomen.

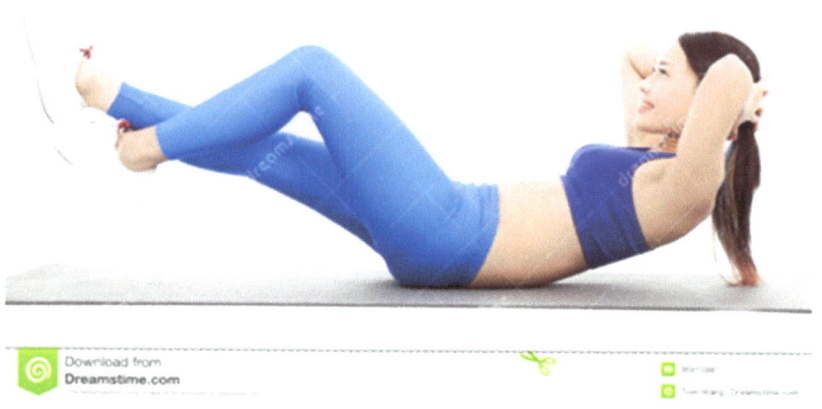

Application

Lie straight on your back on the floor. Take a deep breath and hold your tummy in. Put both hands under your head and hold your head with your hands. Bring your head forward to your chest. Keep your neck and chin straight and breathe out while you lean your chin toward your chest and breathe in while going back. Repeat 10 times for a cycle and give a 30-second break between each cycle.

Benefit

You can literally feel your abdominal muscles working as you squeeze and relax them. It's really good for your upper abdomen, and within months you will find your stomach and upper abdominal muscles going back to their original position.

Dos and Don'ts

Never do this exercise with a full stomach. The best time to do this exercise is in the morning with an empty stomach. Have your breakfast at least an hour after this workout.

EXERCISE 2.

————

Side Crunches

Whether your desk job belittles your leg activity or a lazy lifestyle keeps you away from walking, even if you're too busy with your work and family that you can't take 30 minutes of time out for a relaxing walk, your body has to pay for it. Flabby thighs and love handles look cute on infants only but not on you. The well-toned and trimmed waist with perfect legs can still be obtained if you can incorporate this easy exercise within your daily routine. Side crunches are best for toning your waist and legs.

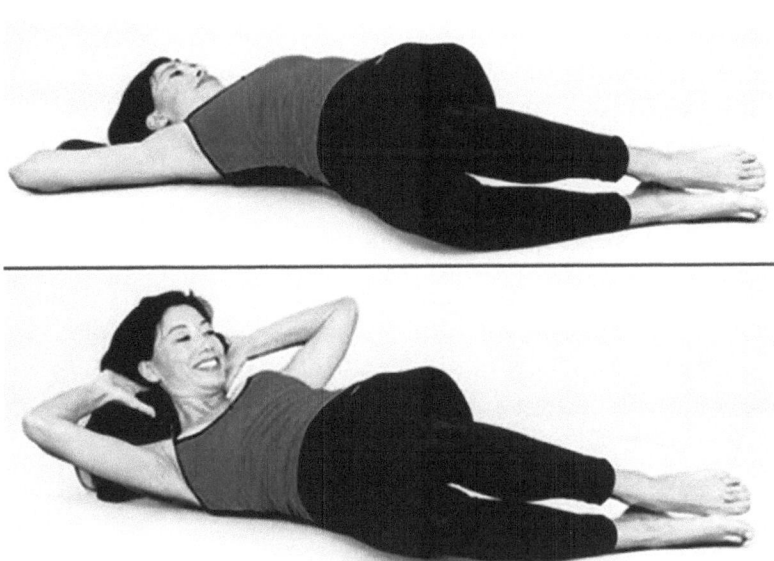

Application

Lie straight in a normal crunch position. Now bend your knees back and turn your legs to one side with your bent knees. Keeping your shoulder blades and upper body flat on the ground, slowly turn your waist. Now lift your head up without bending your neck – just like with a normal crunch. After 1 set of 10 reps, turn your legs to the other side and repeat. Two to 3 sets of this exercise can give you excellent results if done at least 3 times a week.

Benefits

Side crunches not only tone up your thighs and waist but also relax your muscles from strain. This exercise helps in strengthening your waist muscles and maintaining a healthy blood flow to your lower body. You can actually see and feel your lower body muscles working and getting toned up without any extra effort. Consistency is the only requisite!

Dos and Don'ts

Never do the exercise without a warm-up. You can also make it more intense by using an exercise band.

EXERCISE 3.

Best Lower Abdomen Toning Exercise

T his is the most troubled area for women, especially after pregnancy. The muscles loosen up and it looks like a water ball. To get your tummy back in shape, you have to start working on it from day one after your delivery. Here is an easy toning exercise that you can do easily with the help of a chair only.

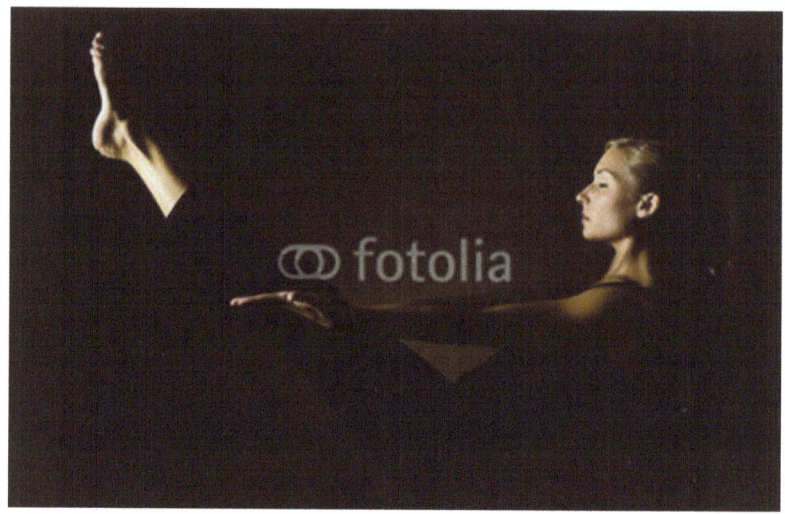

Application

Lie down on the floor in front of a chair that is lower than normal height. Shoulders and back must be flat on the floor while your tummy is tuck in the most you can. Slowly move both legs up only 20 degrees from the ground. Hold it for 30 seconds, keep breathing, and come back down. Do 20 reps per set and 5 sets in your workout.

Once your lower tummy muscles develop enough strength to hold your legs at 20 degrees from the ground, then you raise your legs up to the chair, cross the seat to the right and left. You would feel your lower tummy, thighs, and hips muscles working. Two sets of 15 reps can do the trick.

After this, take 30 seconds to rest and again raise both legs at 20 degrees. Now bend your right knee first and then bend the left knee as you straighten the right – just like you do in cycling. Just remember not to raise your legs higher than 30 degrees.

Benefits

This exercise works wonders on your lower abdomen, thighs, waist, and hips. All those post-pregnancy saggy muscles will actually gain their position back if done with consistency. While the earlier is better, it's never too late and you can start this workout from today and keep it in your routine to gain quicker results.

Dos and Don'ts

Of course, it has to be done with an empty stomach, and that means your last meal should be eaten at least 2 hours before you start this workout. After the workout, you must not drink for half an hour and eat until it's been 1 hour. This exercise lets your abdominal muscles gain strength back and gives better blood flow toward their streams.

EXERCISE 4.

Gaining Back the Trimmed Curves

B ehind those tire tube your smart waist is hidden. Gain it back with this easy toning exercise. No need for sweaty aerobics or other difficult exercises while you can do this simply in the comfort of your home.

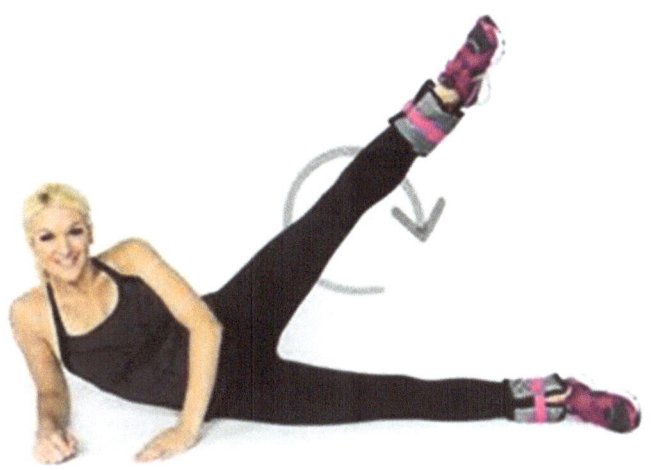

Application

Kneel on the floor and lean all the way over to your right side. Keeping your weight balanced by putting it to the right, slowly raise your left leg to 20-45 degrees from the floor and point your toe and then heel. Knees must be bent forward a little while you raise your leg. Make 8 clockwise circles in the air with your toe and heel. Look out over your hand while bringing the left side of your rib cage toward your hip. Lower to your starting position and repeat 6 to 8 times. Do two sets of 6 to 8 reps, and then switch sides.

Benefits

As you hold up your leg in such a manner, your side muscles stretch and squeeze while making circles in the air. The blood flow to the muscles gets better and fat tissues rupture to give more space to the muscle protein.

This way your side muscle tightens up and forms a toned-up figure.

Dos and Don'ts

You can do this exercise before and after 2 hours of your meal. In the morning before getting up or while watching TV, any time would be suitable. Of course, exercising with a full stomach is not recommended. Also, don't pull up your leg more than 45 degrees, as this is the perfect angle that tends to help your side muscles work with exertion. You can use ankle weights to make it more intense.

EXERCISE 5.

Upper Body Toning

After working out the trickiest lower body parts, here are some of the easiest and best exercises for your neck, shoulders, arms, and breasts. The female body sags more quickly than that of the male; the reasons include pregnancy, breastfeeding, and hormonal cycles. To stay in shape, you can easily do a 10-minute workout that requires nothing but an hour of empty stomach and time.

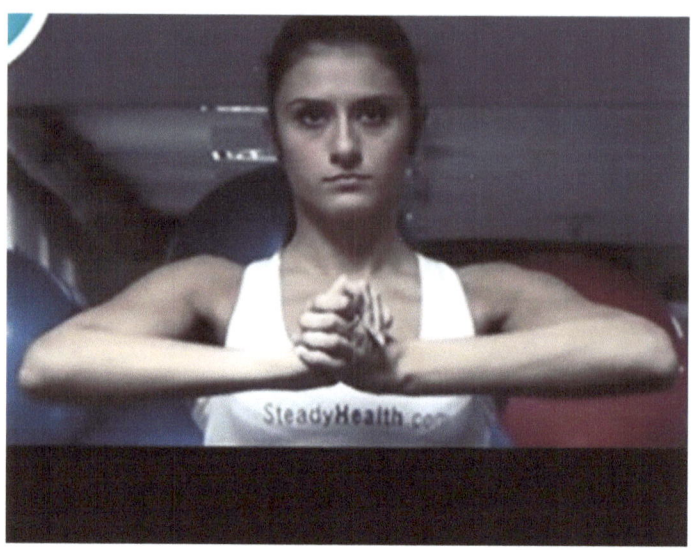

Application

Sit tall on a sturdy chair, shoulder bones straight, and chin balanced. Join both your hands from fingers to elbow in front of your chest. Pull the hands in similar condition upward for 3 seconds and then come back to the same position. Don't undo your hands during the set, and instead keep them steady and firm and repeat. Do 8 cycles in each set and at least 5 set in each workout.

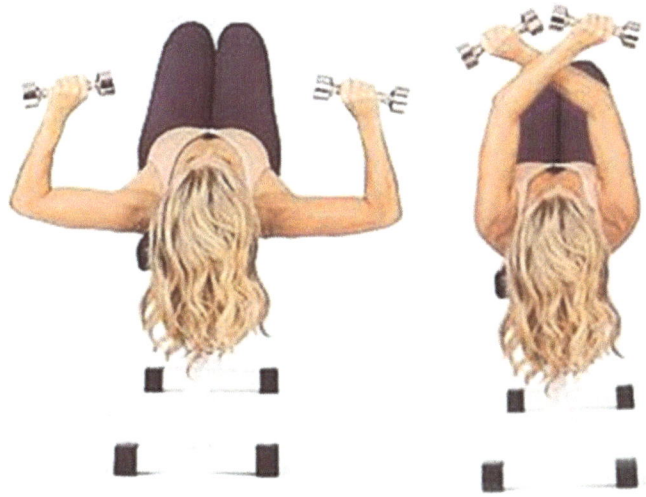

Secondly, take dumbbells or water bottles in your hand. Align them in front of your face. Shoulders and back must be straightened and tummy tucked in, and elbows should be horizontal without any angle. Now move both hands in their own direction until the dumbbells coincide to your ears, then come back. Repeat the cycle for 8 times in a set 2 to 3 sets are recommended in each workout.

Thirdly, hold dumbbells above your shoulders with slightly bent elbows. Keeping them bent, lower the weights until your elbows align with your chest. Keep the same bend as you press the weights up again. This is called a dumbbell fly. Ten reps in a set are recommended.

Dos and Don'ts

The angles of the elbows should be taken seriously. During the whole workout, your back and shoulders must stay straight. Don't forget to breathe. Take deep breaths while performing each exercise.

Benefits

The saggy muscles of the arms, breasts, and ribs get toned up with a consistent workout routine. Gain back your beauty that was lost after giving birth or gaining weight. Stay and look younger than your age. Besides these advantages, your toned-up muscles keep you active and light.

EXERCISE 6.

Bench Press

B ench pressing is the best exercise that can help you remove sagginess from your upper body due the strengthening of the pectoral muscles that support the breast tissue.

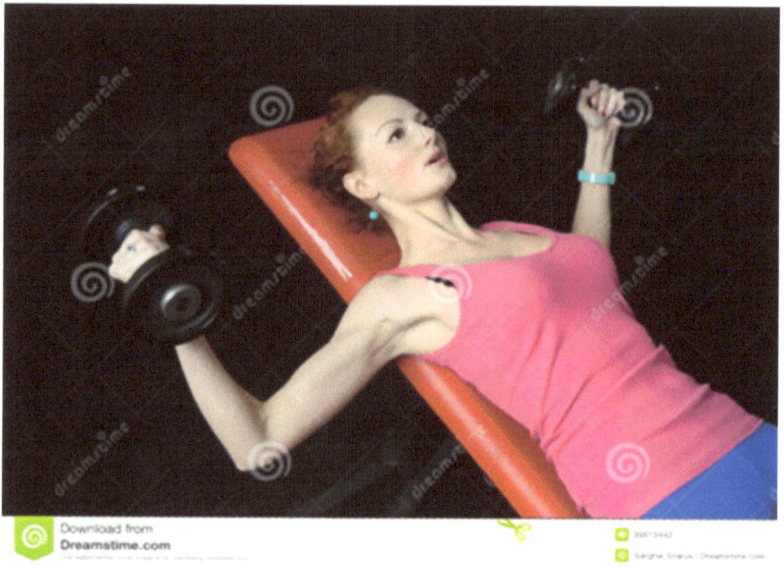

Application

Lie face up on a bench with a dumbbell or water bottle in each hand. Lower the dumbbells until they align with the sides of your chest. Now lift them up straight and then come back again to the starting position. This completes one rep. Do 8 reps in a set. Two-3 sets would do the thing in each workout.

Dos and Don'ts

Don't go beneath your chest limit, as it can cause strain in your muscles. Count 3 seconds in each position and steadily come to the previous position. Don't rush to do the reps. Give it the required time and do it progressively.

Benefits

The bench pressing exercise is well-known for its positive effects. It lifts up the breasts and tones the saggy arm bundles quite successfully. Once you get the desired results, keep this exercise in your regimen in order to maintain the firmness.

EXERCISE 7.

Push-Ups

T he pushup is another great workout for firming your upper body with an added bonus of strengthening your back, arms, and core muscles.

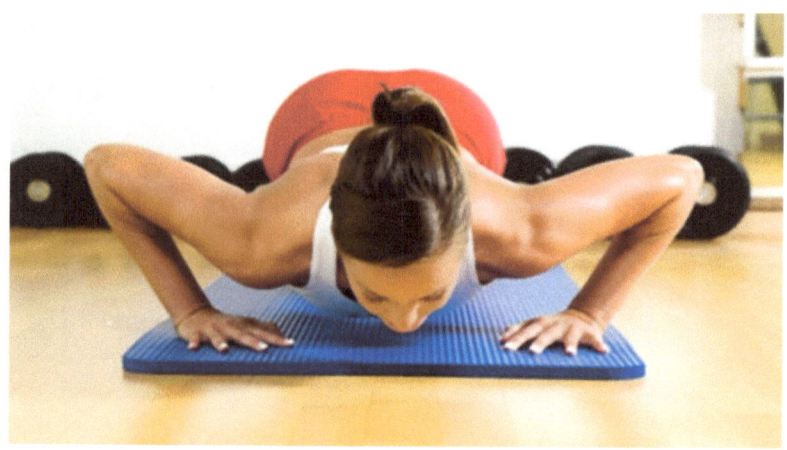

Lie on your tummy on the floor. Put both palms of your hands on the ground opposite to your armpits and tuck your toes inward to the ground. Gradually push your upper body up with the help of your palms, pushing the ground while your elbows are slightly bent. Keep your stomach tucked in. Plank your whole body with a count of ten and then slowly lower your chest to the ground, then push yourself up again. Repeat as many times as you can. If you are looking for a slightly easier version for starters, then you can place your knees on the ground.

Dos and Don'ts

It's better to ask your physician first, especially if you have become a mother recently and if you have stitches. Also, people with excessive weight should start by placing the knees on the ground to avoid muscle strain. The head must be aligned to the spine, and the stomach should be contracted.

Benefits

This exercise is simple but has great effects. It boosts your vigor and stamina. Also, it tones up the whole body without any hassle.

EXERCISE 8.

Chair Crunch

T his move relaxes your muscle tensions and helps in maintaining a straight posture that is seriously balanced and steadier. Confidence boosted! You can also add it with your warm-up as starters.

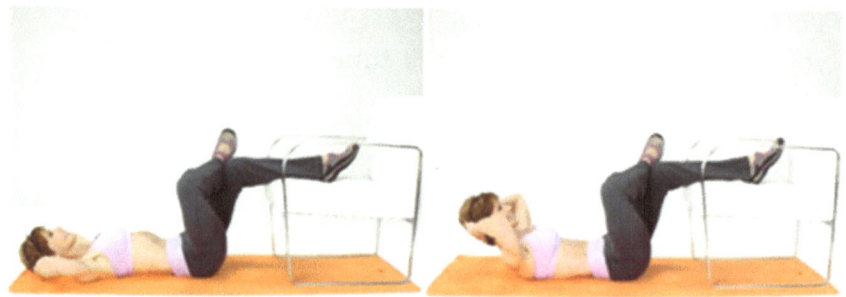

Application

Lie straight on the floor while your legs are on a small chair from toes to knees. Cross your fingers of both hands behind your neck and lean upward so that your left elbow touches your left knee. Repeat the same with your right elbow and right knee. Do 15 to 20 reps with alternating sides too.

Dos and Don'ts

Never use a chair that is not similar in the height of your thighs. You should lie comfortably on the ground, and your back should be aligned with the floor. Pushing up to the knees would be difficult for beginners, so they have to do sets of small reps until they can easily reach their knees.

Benefits

This exercise is great for strengthening your back and abdominal muscles. It brings more flexibility to your muscles and tones them up more rapidly.

EXERCISE 9.

Squat Thrust

A s you gain strength and your knees can handle things more easily, you should try doing squat thrusts, as they work best for toning your back, hips, and thigh muscles.

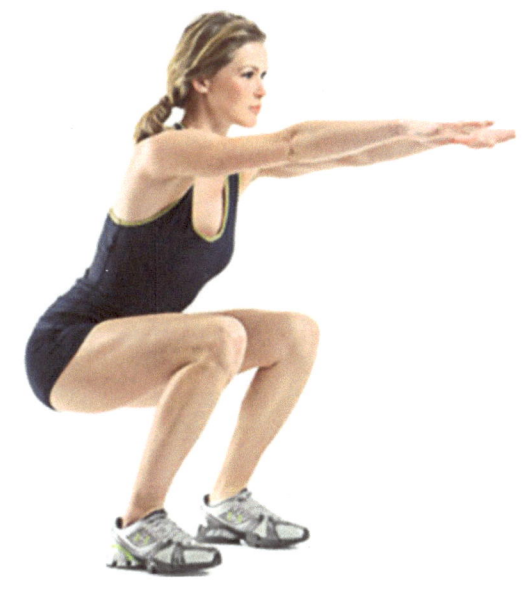

Application

Stand straight with your feet apart to almost shoulder width, and extend your arm in front of you aligned with your shoulder height. To begin the squat, bend your knees to 90 degrees and twist your upper body to the left. Now come up and repeat the process to the right. Keep your knees facing forward as your chest and shoulders move side to side. All your weight should be exerted in your heels, and don't let your knees jut forward away from your toes.

Benefits

The conventional squat thrust sounds tough to most of women, but the added twist can do the trick in an easier way while speeding up the waist-toning process along with the back, thighs, and core. It helps in improving posture, maintaining a center of gravity and balance, along with toning benefits.

Dos and Don'ts

This exercise is not recommended for people who are extremely overweight and new mothers with stitches that have not been removed yet. Also, those who have weak knees should ask their physician first.

EXERCISE 10.

Dead Bug

S tretch and squeeze your tricky zones simultaneously and get a toned figure. This dead bug posture finally covers up your trickiest zones.

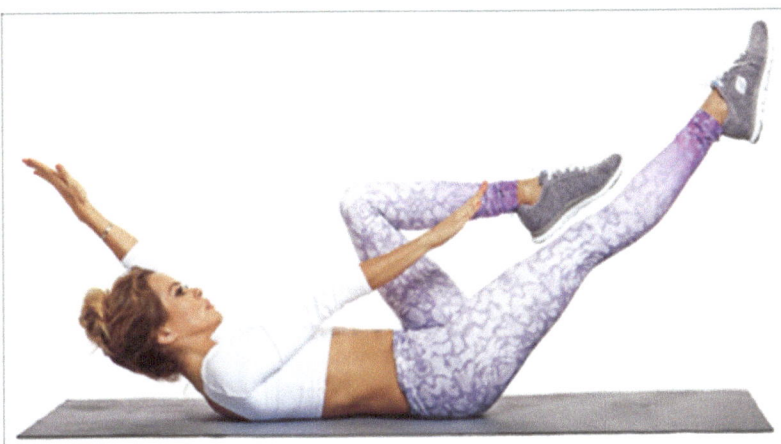

Application

Lie on the floor on your back and bend and raise your knees to a 90-degree angle to the floor. Raise both of your arms up toward the ceiling while keeping your neck, head, and back flat on the floor. Now press your lower back as you exhale deeply. Keep compressing your abs as you extend your right hand behind your head and straighten your left leg. Do the process while keeping your lower back flat on the ground. Repeat the process with the other side. Do 8 reps in each set; 3 sets are recommended for each workout.

BONUS TOPICS

10 things to do for an ache-free workout

Introduction

I t has been said already that health is your first wealth, so never lose it because of your laziness or cravings. The best thing is you can always gain it back with a little bit of effort – depending on your will and efforts. Along with our 10 best ways to tone up your body, you need to focus on following 10 factors to stay in shape and boost your health with positive energy levels.

Just as the holidays are over, I am pretty sure those few more pounds gained from festive dinners must be still lingering. So, it's better to get on track with our recommended toning workouts to avoid muscle soreness and that lazy fat cat feel. Returning back to the routine that hasn't been practiced for over a week tends to cause deferred muscle soreness, as the lactic acid buildup in muscle tissues could take up to at least three days to set in. This could also result in dehydration, cramps, and soreness due to a decrease in blood flow and oxygen to muscle tissues.

When you return to the workout routine that you haven't practiced for weeks, you could also be at an elevated threat of injury, as your muscles are not strong and flexible and not in swift responsive mode. If you try to recover your muscle soreness from a hard workout, you might put your heart muscles in jeopardy. To tackle this, here are some tips on how you can make your workout routine effectual and easy without causing any possible muscle injury. Get back into shape after holidays or the workout lapse and stay healthier.

1. Keep yourself hydrated

Keeping yourself hydrated is the key to avoiding muscle soreness. Especially drink an adequate amount of water before you exercise – not after or when you feel thirsty. A balance of electrolytes and fluids should be maintained before working out. And your muscles will thank you for doing this.

2. Never skip a 10-minute warm-up

Before you jump into any high muscular activity like jogging, brisk walking or playing any game, it's necessary to warm up your body through light warm-up exercises. It helps you get the heart pumping without any difficulty and keeps your muscles warm.

3. Chose a mini-workout rather than full 2 hours of exercise at one time

A full-speed, intense workout or a shorter, 30-minute mentally prepared one – well, going for the second not only saves you time and effort but also keeps the routine adjusted with your daily tasks. The advantages are unlimited. You will experience less discomfort while giving your body chances to develop more flexibility in a steady and gradual way.

4. Interval training

For women, there is never a routine that is steady for long. There are pregnancies, nursing, work, looking after kids and home – surely so many things on their plate. So the intervals between coming back to exercise could be varied according to the factors involved. To counter this issue, you must try interval training. Start with a warm-up and then do a 20-minute workout with intervals of 3 minutes of running and a minute of walking. Repeat until you have done it for twenty minutes.

By doing this, you can stay more energetic while a rise in heart rate has also burned up some fat. Interval training is basically a fat-burning exercise. You can use this technique in other workouts too, such as biking, stair climbing, etc.

5. Cool down

Calming down your body and gradually turning your heart rate back to normal is unavoidable for your system. You must finish your workout with a slow walk or stretching exercise. Muscles can do better stretching when they are still warm, so use this time for some stretching.

6. Mix up different workouts

It's good to reach out from your comfort zone and mix your regular workout routine with some different moves. Do your usual routine one day and something different on another. Balance is the key that can help you decrease the risk of injuries.

7. Setting a goal – seriously!

If you wait for New Year's resolutions and set lofty goals, it will most likely never be accomplished. Just be realistic and think about how you can actually manage to go to the gym five days a week. Most of those who start out this way tend to loosen up and stop eventually.

If you really want to achieve something, start out one or two days a week and stick to this routine for at least a month before adding another day to it.

8. Keep on moving

Shopping and getting groceries or any other activity that needs you to get on your feet for a while is good. And walking or biking to those places and activities are even better. Making exercise a part of your daily life is easy; it leaves the stress out and lets you stay healthier and more active. I wonder what those people are thinking while they drive in their car in rush hour toward the gym – like, seriously!

9. A day's rest a week

Try to take a full day of rest at least every two weeks. It benefits your entire system between workouts, not to mention, it relaxes your muscles and prevents burnout.

10. Eat healthy

Nourish your body with the right kind of fuel. A healthy diet with a proper exercise routine is the best way to sustain a healthy and fit body. Avoid all sugary, processed, and junk food and add organic, proteins, and greens and citrus to your diet. Alcohol and smoking should also be avoided to maintain health and a perfect figure.

CONCLUSION

These easy workouts can enhance your body flexibility, relax your muscles, and tone up your figure without any extra effort. Just take 30 minutes out of your routine and you'll stay younger and healthier for life. Any workout routine has to be done consistently in order to maintain a balanced figure and health. However, this is not possible in a woman's case. They have to switch routines due to certain circumstances that lead to an inconsistent exercise routine. Whenever they get back to their workout regimen, there are some difficulties in the form of muscle soreness, elevated heart rate, and other problems that cause lack of enthusiasm. We have some additional tips and tricks to tackle this issue so that you are always ready for toning, stretching, and routine workouts.

End

OTHER BOOKS BY CARLOS CHAVEZ.

A Healthy Brain: Keeping the Mind Young and Active

by Carlos Chavez.
Link: http://amzn.com/B01ACNZ2LG

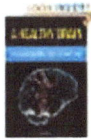

10 Easy Ways to Start Saving Money in 2016: BE MINDFUL WITH YOUR MONEY
by Carlos Chavez
Link: http://amzn.com/B019R1E0PS

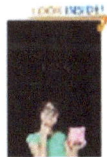

10 Best Ways to Reduce Stress: Easy Techniques to Beat Daily Life Stress
by Carlos Chavez
Link: http://amzn.com/B019O9ZXAY

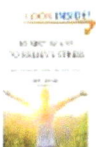

10 Easy Exercises For A Perfectly Toned Body In A Month

CAN I ASK A FAVOR?

If you enjoyed this book, I'd really appreciate it if you would post a short review on Amazon. I do read all the reviews personally so that I can continually write what people are wanting.

If you'd like to leave a review then please visit the link below:

Link: http://amzn.com/B01AOLWLGU

Thanks for your support!

www.ingramcontent.com/pod-product-compliance
Lightning Source LLC
Chambersburg PA
CBHW050843290526
45792CB00002B/506